Ampicillin Usage Manual

A Practical Manual on the Safe Use of
Ampicillin for Treating Bacterial Infections
and Promoting Recovery

Avery Johnston

Legal Notice

Disclaimer

The information presented in this book is provided for educational and informational purposes only. Neither the author nor the publisher is a licensed medical professional, and the content should not be regarded as medical advice. This book is not intended to replace professional medical consultation, diagnosis, or treatment. Always seek the guidance of a qualified healthcare provider regarding any medical questions or concerns.The author and publisher assume no responsibility or liability for any loss, harm, or adverse outcomes resulting from the use or misuse of the information in this book. Readers are solely responsible for any actions taken based on the content provided.

Table of contents

Introduction to Ampicillin

Ampicillin is an antibiotic widely used to treat a range of bacterial infections. As a member of the penicillin family, it is known for its ability to target both gram-positive and some gram-negative bacteria, making it a broad-spectrum antibiotic. However, it is important to note that Ampicillin is only effective against bacterial infections and does not treat viral illnesses, such as the common cold or flu.

This guide provides practical insights into what users need to know about Ampicillin, focusing on safe use, potential risks, and key information to ensure effective treatment.

Ampicillin is a prescription antibiotic that works by interfering with the formation of bacterial cell walls, weakening the bacteria until they can no longer survive. It is commonly prescribed to treat infections affecting the respiratory system, urinary tract, gastrointestinal system, skin, and soft tissues. Additionally, it may be used in the treatment of bacterial meningitis and certain infections caused by Listeria.

Ampicillin can be taken orally in capsules or liquid form, or it can be administered by injection, depending on the type and severity of the infection. Healthcare providers carefully select this medication for specific infections where it has proven to be effective, ensuring that its use is appropriate for each patient's needs.

The primary goal of this guide is to provide users with clear and accurate information about Ampicillin. It aims to answer common questions and outline what individuals need to know to use the medication safely. Key areas covered in the guide include:

How Ampicillin Works: Understanding how the medication targets bacteria.

When to Use Ampicillin: Knowing the types of infections it treats and when it is recommended.

Dosage and Safety Guidelines: Following instructions to ensure effective use and minimize risks.

Managing Side Effects: Identifying common and serious side effects.

Precautions and Drug Interactions: Recognizing situations that require caution.

This guide does not replace professional medical advice but serves as a helpful resource for users to understand what to expect when taking Ampicillin. It emphasizes the importance of consulting a healthcare provider for personalized guidance and encourages adherence to prescribed instructions to achieve the best possible outcome.

Chapter 1

How Ampicillin Works

Ampicillin plays a crucial role in treating bacterial infections by directly targeting the bacteria responsible for illness. Understanding how it works can help users appreciate its effectiveness and the importance of following prescribed instructions. As an antibiotic, Ampicillin doesn't simply relieve symptoms but tackles the root cause of the infection, helping the body recover by eliminating harmful bacteria.

However, like all antibiotics, it is essential to use Ampicillin correctly to ensure it works effectively. This section explains how the medication operates and provides insight into its classification as a broad-spectrum antibiotic.

Mechanism of Action

Ampicillin kills bacteria by disrupting their ability to build protective cell walls. Bacteria rely on their cell walls for structure and protection. Ampicillin interferes with the production of a key component called peptidoglycan, which bacteria need to maintain the integrity of their cell walls.

Without a functional cell wall, bacteria become weak and vulnerable, causing them to burst and die. This process is called bactericidal activity, meaning the drug actively destroys the bacteria, allowing the immune system to complete the healing process.

Since human cells don't have the same type of cell walls as bacteria, Ampicillin specifically targets bacterial cells, making it an effective treatment for infections without harming healthy cells. However, not all bacteria are susceptible to Ampicillin. Some bacteria may resist it by producing enzymes like beta-lactamase, which can break down the antibiotic. That's why healthcare providers may sometimes prescribe it with another drug to enhance its effectiveness.

Understanding Broad-Spectrum Antibiotics

Ampicillin is classified as a broad-spectrum antibiotic because it can target a wide range of bacteria. Specifically, it is effective against:

Gram-positive bacteria, such as Streptococcus and Enterococcus species.

Gram-negative bacteria, including some strains of Escherichia coli and Haemophilus influenzae.

The broad-spectrum nature of Ampicillin makes it a valuable option for treating infections when the exact bacterial cause is unknown, or when multiple types of bacteria may be involved. However, this versatility also comes with responsibilities. Using broad-spectrum antibiotics unnecessarily can contribute to antibiotic resistance, where bacteria adapt and become harder to treat over time.

Healthcare providers are careful to prescribe Ampicillin only when it is necessary, ensuring that it remains effective for treating infections. This is why it's crucial to take the medication exactly as prescribed—finishing the full course, even if symptoms improve early, helps prevent the spread of resistant bacteria.

By understanding how Ampicillin works and the significance of its broad-spectrum capabilities, users can appreciate the importance of using it appropriately. Taking antibiotics responsibly ensures that infections are effectively treated while preserving the power of these medications for future needs.

Chapter 2

Indications for Use of Ampicillin

Ampicillin is a widely utilized antibiotic that belongs to the penicillin group, known for its effectiveness against a variety of bacterial infections. Understanding the indications for its use is crucial for both healthcare providers and patients to ensure appropriate treatment. Ampicillin works by targeting and destroying specific types of bacteria, thereby alleviating the underlying cause of bacterial infections.

This antibiotic is particularly valuable in the treatment of respiratory tract infections, urinary tract infections, gastrointestinal infections, meningitis, listeria infections, and skin and soft tissue infections. However, its use must be guided by the type of infection and the sensitivity of the bacteria involved.

Common Infections Treated with Ampicillin

Ampicillin is indicated for the treatment of several common infections, reflecting its broad-spectrum activity. One of the primary areas where Ampicillin is employed is in the management of respiratory tract infections. Conditions such as pneumonia, which causes inflammation of the lungs, can be effectively treated with this antibiotic. Similarly, bronchitis, an inflammation of the airways, can benefit from Ampicillin's bactericidal properties.

Another significant application of Ampicillin is in treating urinary tract infections (UTIs). These infections, characterized by symptoms such as pain or burning during urination, can often be alleviated by administering Ampicillin, especially when the bacteria involved are known to be susceptible to the medication.

In the gastrointestinal tract, Ampicillin is effective against infections caused by bacteria such as Salmonella and Shigella, which can lead to severe gastrointestinal distress and dehydration. Furthermore, Ampicillin is utilized in the treatment of bacterial meningitis, a serious condition that necessitates prompt and effective antibiotic therapy to prevent severe complications.

Moreover, Ampicillin is also used to treat infections caused by Listeria monocytogenes, particularly in vulnerable populations such as pregnant women and newborns. In addition to these infections, Ampicillin plays a role in managing skin and soft tissue infections, such as cellulitis, where bacteria enter the skin through cuts or abrasions.

When Ampicillin May Be Recommended

The decision to prescribe Ampicillin is based on several critical factors. Firstly, laboratory tests are often conducted to confirm the bacterial strain causing the infection and to determine its susceptibility to Ampicillin. If the bacteria are confirmed to be sensitive, healthcare providers may recommend this antibiotic as a suitable treatment option.

Furthermore, Ampicillin's broad-spectrum nature makes it an excellent choice when there is a need for coverage against multiple types of bacteria, particularly when the specific cause of the infection is not immediately identifiable. This versatility allows healthcare providers to address infections effectively without delay.

In cases where patients cannot tolerate alternative antibiotics due to allergies or adverse reactions, Ampicillin may be recommended as a viable option. Additionally, in certain situations, Ampicillin is utilized prophylactically to prevent infections, especially in surgical patients or those with weakened immune systems.

Lastly, Ampicillin may be prescribed to manage infections that occur during pregnancy, such as group B streptococcus, to protect both the mother and the developing fetus from potential complications.

In conclusion, Ampicillin is a critical antibiotic with well-defined indications for use, targeting various bacterial infections effectively. Understanding its applications and the circumstances under which it is prescribed can help ensure its responsible use, ultimately enhancing patient outcomes and combating the spread of antibiotic resistance. By adhering to healthcare provider recommendations, individuals can contribute to the successful treatment of infections while minimizing potential risks associated with antibiotic use.

Chapter 3

Dosage and Administration of Ampicillin

The proper dosage and administration of Ampicillin are essential for maximizing its effectiveness and minimizing the risk of side effects. Understanding the recommended dosages for different age groups, the various methods of administration, and what to do in case of missed doses is crucial for anyone using this antibiotic.

Recommended Dosages for Adults and Children

Ampicillin dosage varies depending on the type and severity of the infection being treated, as well as the age and weight of the patient. For adults, the typical dosage ranges from 250 mg to 500 mg every 6 hours, or 1 g every 8 hours, depending on the specific infection. In more severe cases, the healthcare provider may increase the dosage to 2 g every 4 to 6 hours.

For children, the dosage is usually based on their weight. The general recommendation is 50 to 100 mg per kilogram of body weight per day, divided into several doses. For serious infections, such as meningitis, higher dosages may be prescribed, sometimes reaching up to 300 mg per kilogram of body weight. It's important for caregivers to consult with a healthcare professional to determine the appropriate dosage tailored to the child's individual needs.

In all cases, adherence to the prescribed dosage is vital. Taking more than the recommended dose can lead to increased side effects and potential toxicity, while under-dosing may result in ineffective treatment and the risk of developing antibiotic-resistant bacteria.

Methods of Administration (Oral vs. Injection)

Ampicillin can be administered through different routes, with the most common being oral and intravenous (IV) injection. The choice of administration method typically depends on the severity of the infection and the patient's condition.

1. Oral Administration:

Ampicillin is available in capsule and liquid forms for oral intake. It is usually taken with or without food, although taking it with food may help reduce potential gastrointestinal discomfort. For optimal absorption, it is recommended to avoid taking it simultaneously with antacids or other medications containing iron or calcium.

2. Injection:

For more serious infections or when a rapid therapeutic effect is needed, Ampicillin may be administered via intravenous (IV) injection. This method allows for direct delivery into the bloodstream, ensuring that the drug reaches the site of infection quickly. Healthcare providers typically determine the specific route and method of administration based on the patient's needs and clinical judgment.

Patients should follow healthcare providers' instructions regarding the method of administration to ensure the most effective treatment.

Instructions for Missed Doses

Missed doses can happen, but knowing how to manage them is important for maintaining effective treatment. If a dose of Ampicillin is missed, the patient should take it as soon as they remember. However, if it is almost time for the next scheduled dose, they should skip the missed dose and continue with the regular dosing schedule.

Patients should never double the dose to catch up, as this can increase the risk of side effects and may lead to complications. For those on a strict schedule or those who have questions about managing missed doses, consulting with a healthcare provider is always advisable.

In summary, understanding the recommended dosages, administration methods, and handling missed doses of Ampicillin is crucial for ensuring the antibiotic's effectiveness while minimizing potential risks. Patients should always follow healthcare provider recommendations and guidelines for the best outcomes in their treatment.

Chapter 4

Precautions and Warnings for Ampicillin

Ampicillin is a powerful antibiotic with a wide range of applications in treating bacterial infections. However, like all medications, it is essential to be aware of the precautions and warnings associated with its use to ensure safe and effective treatment. This section discusses situations requiring caution, contraindications, and considerations for special populations.

Situations Requiring Caution

Patients should exercise caution when using Ampicillin in certain circumstances. One of the most critical considerations is the presence of allergies. Individuals with a known allergy to penicillin or other beta-lactam antibiotics should inform their healthcare provider before starting Ampicillin, as severe allergic reactions can occur. Symptoms of an allergic reaction may include hives, difficulty breathing, and swelling of the face or throat. In such cases, alternative antibiotics may be considered to avoid potential complications.

Additionally, patients with a history of asthma, hay fever, or hives may be at an increased risk of allergic reactions to Ampicillin. It is essential to discuss any previous allergic reactions with a healthcare provider to ensure safe prescribing practices.

Furthermore, individuals with kidney disease or impaired renal function should use Ampicillin with caution, as the drug is primarily excreted through the kidneys. In such patients, dosages may need to be adjusted to prevent toxicity and adverse effects.

Contraindications: When Not to Use Ampicillin

Ampicillin should not be used in specific situations where its use may pose more risks than benefits. The most significant contraindication is in patients with a known hypersensitivity to penicillin or any component of the formulation. As mentioned earlier, such individuals are at risk of severe allergic reactions, making it unsafe for them to take Ampicillin.

Moreover, Ampicillin should be used cautiously in patients with a history of cholestatic jaundice or hepatic dysfunction related to prior use of penicillins. In these cases, using Ampicillin could lead to further liver complications, and alternative treatments may be more appropriate.

Lastly, Ampicillin is contraindicated in certain cases of infectious mononucleosis, as its use in these patients can lead to a rash that may be misinterpreted as an allergic reaction, complicating the clinical picture.

Use in Special Populations

Ampicillin's use may vary in special populations, including pregnant individuals, breastfeeding mothers, the elderly, and pediatric patients. Understanding these nuances is vital for ensuring safe and effective treatment.

1. Pregnant Individuals:

Ampicillin is generally considered safe for use during pregnancy when prescribed by a healthcare provider. It has been classified as a Category B medication, meaning there is no evidence of harm to the fetus in animal studies. However, pregnant individuals should always discuss the potential risks and benefits with their healthcare provider to make informed decisions.

2. Breastfeeding:

Ampicillin is excreted in breast milk in small amounts. While it is typically deemed safe for breastfeeding mothers, it is essential to monitor the infant for potential side effects, such as gastrointestinal upset or allergic reactions. Consulting a healthcare provider before using Ampicillin while breastfeeding is advisable to address any concerns.

3. Elderly Patients:

Older adults may be more susceptible to the side effects of Ampicillin due to potential age-related changes in kidney function. Healthcare providers may adjust the dosage accordingly to minimize the risk of adverse reactions and ensure effective treatment.

4. Pediatric Patients:

Ampicillin can be prescribed to children, but dosage is usually determined based on the child's weight and age. Caregivers should ensure that the medication is administered as prescribed and monitor for any side effects or allergic reactions.

In conclusion, while Ampicillin is an effective antibiotic for treating various bacterial infections, it is vital to be aware of the precautions and warnings associated with its use. By understanding situations that require caution, recognizing contraindications, and considering the unique needs of special populations, patients and healthcare providers can work together to ensure safe and effective treatment outcomes. Always consult with a healthcare professional before starting or adjusting any medication regimen.

Chapter 5

Potential Side Effects of Ampicillin

While Ampicillin is an effective antibiotic used to treat various bacterial infections, it may also cause side effects. Understanding these potential effects, both common and serious, is essential for anyone taking this medication. Being informed helps users manage side effects appropriately and know when to seek medical attention.

Common Side Effects and How to Manage Them

Many patients may experience mild to moderate side effects while taking Ampicillin. Common side effects include:

1. Gastrointestinal Issues:

Symptoms: Nausea, vomiting, diarrhea, and abdominal discomfort are frequently reported.

Management: Taking Ampicillin with food may help alleviate some gastrointestinal upset. Staying hydrated is important, especially if diarrhea occurs. Over-the-counter medications, such as loperamide, can be used for diarrhea, but it is wise to consult a healthcare provider before using them, especially in cases of severe diarrhea.

2. **Allergic Reactions:**

Symptoms: Mild rashes or itching may occur, particularly in individuals with allergies to penicillin.

Management: Over-the-counter antihistamines can help manage mild allergic reactions. However, if symptoms worsen or if hives or swelling develops, it's important to seek medical attention immediately.

3. Yeast Infections:

Symptoms: Antibiotics like Ampicillin can disrupt the natural balance of bacteria in the body, potentially leading to yeast infections.

Management: Maintaining good hygiene and, if necessary, discussing the use of antifungal treatments with a healthcare provider can help manage this side effect.

4. Headaches:

Symptoms: Some individuals may experience headaches while taking Ampicillin.

Management: Staying well-hydrated and using over-the-counter pain relievers, like acetaminophen or ibuprofen, may provide relief.

While these common side effects may be bothersome, they are generally not serious and can often be managed with simple remedies.

Recognizing Serious Adverse Reactions

Although rare, some individuals may experience serious side effects that require immediate medical attention. Recognizing these reactions is crucial:

1.Severe Allergic Reactions (Anaphylaxis):

Symptoms: Difficulty breathing, swelling of the face or throat, rapid heartbeat, and severe dizziness.

Action: This is a medical emergency. Call emergency services or seek immediate medical care.

2. Clostridium difficile Infection:

Symptoms: Severe diarrhea, abdominal cramps, and fever. This infection can occur after antibiotic use due to disruption of gut bacteria.

Action: Contact a healthcare provider if these symptoms develop, as this condition may require specific treatment.

3. Liver Issues:

Symptoms: Yellowing of the skin or eyes (jaundice), dark urine, or severe fatigue.

Action: Report these symptoms to a healthcare provider, as they may indicate liver dysfunction.

4. Severe Skin Reactions:

Symptoms: Blistering, peeling, or red skin rashes that spread rapidly.

Action: Seek immediate medical attention if you experience any of these symptoms.

When to Contact a Healthcare Provider

Patients should maintain open communication with their healthcare providers while taking Ampicillin. It is essential to contact a healthcare provider if:

Common side effects persist or worsen, causing significant discomfort.

Symptoms of an allergic reaction occur, even if mild.

Any serious adverse reactions are suspected, as outlined above.

There are concerns about the effectiveness of the treatment, or if symptoms of the infection do not improve within a few days.

Being proactive about health and recognizing the signs of potential side effects can lead to more effective management and ensure safe treatment with Ampicillin. Patients are encouraged to keep their healthcare provider informed of any new or unusual symptoms they may experience during their treatment.

Chapter 6

Drug Interactions with Ampicillin

Understanding drug interactions is crucial when taking any medication, including Ampicillin. Interactions can affect how the drug works or increase the risk of side effects. This section outlines medications that may interact with Ampicillin, discusses its impact on birth control effectiveness, and provides tips on minimizing interaction risks.

Medications That May Interact with Ampicillin

Several medications can interact with Ampicillin, potentially altering its effectiveness or increasing the risk of adverse effects. Some key interactions to be aware of include:

1. Probenecid:

Description: Often used to treat gout, probenecid can inhibit the renal excretion of Ampicillin.

Impact: This may increase Ampicillin levels in the bloodstream, leading to a higher risk of side effects. If you are prescribed both medications, your healthcare provider may adjust the dosages accordingly.

2. Anticoagulants (e.g., Warfarin):

Description: These medications are used to prevent blood clots.

Impact: Ampicillin may enhance the anticoagulant effect of drugs like warfarin, increasing the risk of bleeding. Regular monitoring of blood clotting parameters is essential when these medications are used together.

3. Other Antibiotics:

Description: Using multiple antibiotics simultaneously can lead to competition for bacterial targets or increased side effects.

Impact: Certain antibiotics, such as tetracyclines or aminoglycosides, may interfere with Ampicillin's effectiveness. Always inform your healthcare provider of all medications you are taking to avoid unnecessary combinations.

4. Methotrexate:

Description: Used to treat certain cancers and autoimmune diseases, methotrexate can interact with many medications.

Impact: Ampicillin may reduce the excretion of methotrexate, potentially leading to toxic levels. Healthcare providers should carefully monitor patients on both medications.

Impact on Birth Control Effectiveness

There is a common concern regarding the use of antibiotics and their impact on hormonal birth control methods. While Ampicillin is not known to significantly reduce the effectiveness of hormonal contraceptives like the pill, patch, or ring, some anecdotal reports suggest that certain antibiotics might interact with contraceptive efficacy.

1. Research Findings:

Most studies indicate that Ampicillin and other penicillin antibiotics do not have a clinically significant impact on the effectiveness of hormonal birth control. However, it is essential to consider that gastrointestinal side effects, such as vomiting or diarrhea, which can occur with

Ampicillin, may impair the absorption of the contraceptive.

2. Recommendation:

If you are taking hormonal birth control and are prescribed Ampicillin, discuss with your healthcare provider whether additional contraceptive methods should be employed during and shortly after the course of treatment, especially if you experience gastrointestinal disturbances.

How to Minimize Interaction Risks

To ensure safe and effective treatment with Ampicillin, consider the following strategies to minimize the risks of drug interactions:

1. Inform Your Healthcare Provider:

Always disclose all medications, supplements, and over-the-counter drugs you are taking to your healthcare provider. This information is critical for assessing potential interactions and making informed prescribing decisions.

2. Follow Prescribing Guidelines:

Adhere strictly to your healthcare provider's instructions regarding the dosage and timing of Ampicillin. Do not modify your medication regimen without consulting your provider, especially if you are taking other medications.

3. Monitor for Side Effects:

Be vigilant about any unusual symptoms or side effects while taking Ampicillin, especially if you are on multiple medications. Report any changes to your healthcare provider promptly.

4. Avoid Self-Medicating:

Refrain from adding new medications or supplements without consulting your healthcare provider. This includes herbal products, which can also interact with prescribed medications.

5. Regular Check-Ups:

Schedule regular follow-ups with your healthcare provider to assess the effectiveness of Ampicillin and monitor for any potential drug interactions, especially if you have complex health needs or are on multiple medications.

In conclusion, while Ampicillin is a valuable tool in treating bacterial infections, being informed about potential drug interactions is crucial for ensuring safe use. By understanding which medications may interact with Ampicillin, the implications for birth control effectiveness, and how to minimize risks, patients can help optimize their treatment outcomes and maintain their health. Always consult with your healthcare provider for personalized advice and recommendations regarding your medication regimen.

Chapter 7

Guidelines for Safe Use of Ampicillin

Ensuring the safe and effective use of Ampicillin is essential for achieving the best outcomes while minimizing risks. This section provides guidelines on proper storage and handling, tips for the safe disposal of unused medication, and strategies for avoiding antibiotic resistance.

Proper Storage and Handling

Proper storage of Ampicillin is crucial to maintain its efficacy and ensure patient safety. Here are some key guidelines:

1. Temperature Control:

Ampicillin should be stored at room temperature, away from excessive heat or moisture. Avoid leaving it in places like bathrooms, where humidity may affect the medication's stability.

2. Keep Out of Reach of Children:

Store Ampicillin in a secure location, out of the reach of children and pets. Accidental ingestion of antibiotics can be dangerous, leading to potential side effects and misuse.

3. Check Expiration Dates:

Regularly check the expiration date on the medication packaging. Do not use Ampicillin past its expiration date, as it may not be effective and could pose health risks.

4. Packaging Integrity:

Ensure that the medication's packaging is intact. If there are any signs of damage, such as broken seals or unusual discoloration, consult your pharmacist or healthcare provider before use.

Tips for Safe Disposal of Unused Medication

Improper disposal of unused medications can pose environmental hazards and risks to public health. Here are some safe disposal tips:

1. Take-Back Programs:

Participate in community drug take-back programs or events, which are often organized by pharmacies, local health departments, or law enforcement agencies. These programs allow for safe disposal of unused medications.

2. Disposal in Household Trash:

If a take-back program is not available, you can dispose of Ampicillin in the household trash by following these steps:

Mix the medication (do not crush tablets or capsules) with an undesirable substance, such as used coffee grounds or cat litter, to make it less appealing to children and pets.

Place the mixture in a sealed plastic bag or container to prevent leakage.

Dispose of the container in your household trash.

3. Flushing:

Flushing medications down the toilet is not generally recommended, as it can contribute to water pollution. However, if the medication label or patient information specifically advises flushing, you should follow those instructions.

4. Remove Personal Information:

Before disposing of any medication containers, be sure to remove or scratch out any personal information, including your name and prescription number, to protect your privacy.

Avoiding Antibiotic Resistance

Antibiotic resistance is a growing public health concern, and responsible use of antibiotics like Ampicillin is essential in combating this issue. Here are some strategies to minimize the risk of developing antibiotic resistance:

1. Take Only as Prescribed:

Use Ampicillin only when prescribed by a healthcare provider and follow the prescribed dosage and duration. Do not skip doses or stop taking the medication prematurely, even if symptoms improve. Completing the full course helps eliminate the bacteria and reduces the risk of resistance.

2. Do Not Share Antibiotics:

Never share Ampicillin or any antibiotics with others, even if they have similar symptoms. Each infection is unique, and only a healthcare provider can determine the appropriate treatment for a specific condition.

3. Avoid Self-Medicating:

Do not use leftover antibiotics from previous treatments or purchase antibiotics without a prescription. Self-medicating can lead to inappropriate use, increasing the risk of resistance.

4. Practice Good Hygiene:

Maintain good hygiene practices, such as regular handwashing and proper food handling, to reduce the risk of infections. Fewer infections mean less reliance on antibiotics, helping to prevent resistance.

5. Stay Informed:

Educate yourself and others about antibiotic resistance and the importance of responsible antibiotic use. Awareness can lead to better practices in both personal and community health.

In conclusion, following these guidelines for the safe use of Ampicillin will help ensure effective treatment while minimizing risks to both individual health and public safety. Proper storage and disposal practices, combined with a commitment to responsible antibiotic use, can significantly contribute to combating antibiotic resistance and safeguarding the effectiveness of antibiotics for future generations. Always consult your healthcare provider with any questions or concerns regarding the use of Ampicillin or other medications.

Chapter 8

frequently Asked Questions (FAQs) About Ampicillin

When taking Ampicillin, patients often have questions regarding its use, effects, and what to expect during treatment. This section addresses common queries to provide clarity and guidance while ensuring the information is accurate and not misleading.

What to Expect During Treatment

When beginning treatment with Ampicillin, it's essential to understand what to expect. Here are some key points:

1. Initial Response:

Many patients may start to feel relief from symptoms within a few days of starting Ampicillin. However, it is crucial to continue taking the medication as prescribed, even if symptoms improve, to ensure that the infection is fully eradicated.

2. Possible Side Effects:

As with any medication, some individuals may experience side effects while taking Ampicillin. Common side effects can include nausea, diarrhea, and mild skin rashes. Most side effects are generally mild and may resolve as your body adjusts to the medication. However, if you experience severe side effects or symptoms such as difficulty breathing, swelling, or a rash, seek medical attention immediately.

3. Follow-Up:

Depending on the type and severity of the infection, your healthcare provider may schedule follow-up appointments to monitor your progress and ensure the infection is responding to treatment. It's essential to attend these appointments and discuss any concerns or questions you may have about your treatment.

Can I Drink Alcohol While Taking Ampicillin?

Alcohol consumption during antibiotic treatment is a common concern among patients. Here's what you should know about drinking alcohol while taking Ampicillin:

1. No Major Interactions:

While moderate alcohol consumption is generally considered safe when taking Ampicillin, it is still advisable to limit or avoid alcohol. This is because alcohol can exacerbate certain side effects of antibiotics, such as stomach upset and dizziness, making it harder for the body to recover from an infection.

2. Impact on Recovery:

Drinking alcohol can also affect your immune system and overall recovery process. Since Ampicillin is used to treat bacterial infections, it's best to allow your body the best chance to heal without the potential interference from alcohol.

3. Consult Your Healthcare Provider:

If you have specific concerns about alcohol consumption while taking Ampicillin or if you have underlying health conditions that may be affected by alcohol, it's essential to discuss this with your healthcare provider for personalized advice.

How Long Does Ampicillin Take to Work?

The time it takes for Ampicillin to start working can vary depending on several factors, including the type of infection being treated and individual patient response. Here are some points to consider:

1. Initial Improvement:

Many patients may begin to notice an improvement in symptoms within 24 to 72 hours after starting treatment with Ampicillin. However, this does not mean the infection is fully cleared, so it is vital to complete the prescribed course.

2. Full Course Duration:

The complete course of Ampicillin typically lasts from 7 to 14 days, depending on the specific infection being treated. It's important to adhere to your healthcare provider's prescribed duration, as stopping treatment early can lead to incomplete eradication of the bacteria and increase the risk of developing antibiotic resistance.

3. Individual Variability:

Factors such as the severity of the infection, the patient's overall health, and adherence to the prescribed dosage can all influence how quickly Ampicillin works. If you do not notice any improvement in your symptoms after a few days of treatment, or if symptoms worsen, contact your healthcare provider for further evaluation.

In conclusion, understanding these frequently asked questions about Ampicillin can help alleviate concerns and enhance patient compliance during treatment. Always consult your healthcare provider with any additional questions or concerns regarding your specific situation to ensure safe and effective use of Ampicillin.

Chapter 9

Monitoring During Treatment with Ampicillin

Monitoring during treatment is essential to ensure the effectiveness of Ampicillin and to identify any potential complications or need for adjustments. This section covers key aspects of monitoring, including follow-up appointments, recognizing treatment outcomes, and considerations for patients with kidney or liver conditions.

Follow-up with Healthcare Providers

Regular follow-up appointments with your healthcare provider are crucial during treatment with Ampicillin. Here's what you need to know:

1. Schedule Regular Appointments:

Follow-up visits allow your healthcare provider to assess your progress and determine whether the Ampicillin is effectively treating your infection. It's essential to keep these appointments as scheduled, even if you start to feel better.

2. Monitoring Symptoms:

During follow-ups, your healthcare provider will ask about any changes in your symptoms. Be prepared to discuss how you feel, any side effects you may be experiencing, and whether there has been an improvement in your condition.

3. Additional Tests:

In some cases, your healthcare provider may recommend laboratory tests, such as blood tests or cultures, to evaluate the effectiveness of the treatment and monitor for any complications. These tests can help ensure that the infection is responding to

Ampicillin and that no new issues have arisen.

3. Importance of Communication:

Maintaining open communication with your healthcare provider is key. Discuss any concerns or changes in your condition as soon as they arise to facilitate timely adjustments to your treatment plan if necessary.

Adjustments for Kidney or Liver Conditions

Patients with pre-existing kidney or liver conditions may require special consideration during treatment with Ampicillin. Here's what to keep in mind:

1. Impact of Kidney Function:

Ampicillin is primarily excreted through the kidneys. If you have impaired kidney function, your healthcare provider may need to adjust your dosage or monitor your kidney function more closely to avoid potential toxicity.

2. Liver Function Considerations:

While Ampicillin is not extensively metabolized by the liver, patients with liver impairment should still be monitored closely. If you have liver conditions, inform your healthcare provider, as they may consider alternative treatments or require additional monitoring.

3. Personalized Treatment Plans:

It's essential to work closely with your healthcare provider to create a personalized treatment plan that considers your kidney and liver health. Regular monitoring may include blood tests to assess kidney and liver function, ensuring that treatment remains safe and effective.

In conclusion, monitoring during treatment with Ampicillin is vital for ensuring optimal outcomes and minimizing risks. Regular follow-up appointments, recognizing treatment success or failure, and adjusting for kidney or liver conditions are crucial components of effective management. Always communicate openly with your healthcare provider and report any changes in your condition to ensure the best possible care throughout your treatment journey.

Conclusion

In conclusion, the safe and effective use of Ampicillin is paramount for successfully treating bacterial infections. Patients must understand the importance of adhering to the prescribed dosage and treatment duration to ensure the complete eradication of the infection and to prevent the development of antibiotic resistance.

Completing the full course of antibiotics, even if symptoms improve before finishing the medication, is crucial to minimize the risk of recurrence and safeguard overall health. Open communication with healthcare providers is essential for addressing any concerns or side effects during treatment. By prioritizing these practices, patients can enhance their treatment outcomes and contribute to a broader effort in managing public health concerns related to antibiotic use.

Made in the USA
Coppell, TX
17 December 2024

42865435R00039